¡MENTAL!
IN THE TRUMP ERA

Ten Inspirational Stories About
Immigrants Overcoming Addiction,
Depression and Anxiety in America

By

Pierluigi Mancini, PhD

Foreword by Sergio Aguilar-Gaxiola, MD, PhD

Copyright © 2018 by Pierluigi Mancini PhD
All rights reserved.

ISBN-13: 978-1987762976
ISBN-10: 1987762975

Dedication

I dedicate this book to all the suffering and recovering addicts, alcoholics, mentally ill individuals, their family members, caregivers and everyone in support of their care.

I also dedicate this book to my loving wife Robin, my daughter Gabriella and my son Julian who have given me more than a purpose to live.

To my father Giovanni, may he rest in peace, and my mother Gladys who continues to teach me every day about love, faith and family and the true meaning of the word 'unconditional'.

And finally my brothers, Giovanni, Aldo, Fabrizio and Paolo who have remained the strongest part of my foundation, the rocks I can always lean on.

Thank you for all you do for me.

Table of Contents

Foreword - Sergio Aguilar-Gaxiola, MD, PhD i

Insight from my own recovery journey iv

Responding to the Needs of Immigrants x

Chapters

1. Chapter 1 – Carolina's solution to Psychosis and Anxiety 1
2. Chapter 2 – Eduardo's solution to Alcoholism, Panic and Anxiety 9
3. Chapter 3 – Carlos' solution for Impulse Control and Marijuana 13
4. Chapter 4 – Estella's solution to Bipolar Disorder and Anxiety Solution 18
5. Chapter 5 – Rosa's solution to Obsession and Depression Solutions 23
6. Chapter 6 – Ofelia's solution to Anxiety and Mood Disorders 28
7. Chapter 7 – Johnny's solution to Substance Use Disorder and Oppositional Defiant Disorder 33
8. Chapter 8 – Alana's solution to Depression and Post Traumatic Stress Disorder 38
9. Chapter 9 – Laura's solution to Depression and Anxiety 43
10. Chapter 10 – Roberto's solution to Schizophrenia 49

Appendix

- Definition of Counseling Services Mentioned in this Book 56
- Dr. Mancini's recommended assessment tools 57

Foreword

This book is a breath of fresh air for it contains eleven powerful personal stories of the journey immigrants from Latin America have gone through and the mental health challenges they have faced. These remarkable and resilient human beings have been hurt with various mental health conditions. However, through hard work, determination, a sense of purpose, and hope they have overcome the overwhelming odds of living in despair. They all share with the readers practical lessons learned and solutions to the predicaments they once found themselves in.

The first pages, which introduce us to Dr. Pierluigi Mancini's journey, result from his life experiences during his young adult life when his addiction struggles became disabling and the beginning of his journey toward recovery. Pierluigi's story, capturing not only his vulnerability to substance use, but also his courage and resilience to seek and find his recovery, represents the power of human lived experiences in giving meaning and authenticity to a much-needed dialogue about mental health challenges and solutions to achieving health equality among our most vulnerable immigrant communities in the United States.

Pierluigi's book admirably sheds light to an issue that continues to impact the lives of Latino immigrants and other underserved communities—the lack of culturally and linguistically appropriate treatment. "It reminded me of how difficult it was for my mother, who was bilingual, to fully understand and be able to communicate with clinicians who did not understand the cultural frame from which she was coming [from]" recalls Pierluigi when seeing the only Latino accessing services after 15 years working in an Atlanta clinic.

Pierluigi's journey from his struggles with comorbid conditions (substance use and mental illness) to starting his own clinic tailored for the cultural and language needs of Latinos and immigrants is inspiring and offers one simple yet powerful message, "Recovery and quality of life is possible." Pierluigi's lived experiences combined with the profound human stories of peoples' journeys toward recovery, and his passion to bringing vulnerable communities out of the shadow and giving them a voice is the impetus of his book. Pierluigi also calls on the future workforce and organizations to confront the bigotry that immigrant populations often face, and work together to collectively defeat the stigma associated with addiction and mental illness.

This volume of stories may provoke mixed reactions from some readers. Some will deem these stories as simply supporting "illegals and criminals" who are mooching off of tax-paying Americans, overburdening the health care system, blah, blah, blah. Others will simply miss the poignant point that if we want to improve quality of care and quality of life for ALL communities, we cannot afford to leave the most vulnerable communities behind and risk the prosperity and well-being of all communities.

Pierluigi brings to light the current political climate where we are seeing progress toward unauthorized individuals and families having access to appropriate mental health care give way to fear, anxiety, isolation, and hopelessness. The same type of hopelessness that Paulo Freire[1] describes as "a form of silence, of denying the world and fleeing from it." Under the Trump administration, we have already seen the negative consequences of adults and children fearing and isolating themselves from participating in community and everyday activities to avoid being targeted for deportation. For example, immigrants and mixed-status families who desperately need help won't seek it out of fear of deportation and exposing other unauthorized family members. These negative consequences increase stigma, distrust, and expose already vulnerable communities to more trauma, prolonged suffering, and other risk factors associated with mental illness.

The theme that all ten stories have in common is this belief that continuing to fight every day and remain resilient in the face of new challenges strengthens one's hope. It was this hope that put these individuals and their families on a path toward recovery. These stories describing their interactions with the mental health system brings us back to Pierluigi's story and his "Recovery and quality of life is possible" blueprint. A recovery blueprint that calls us and our vocation to better serve those in need by creating a system and workforce that is culturally and linguistically appropriate.

That same recovery blueprint gave Carolina the hope that she needed to stay and persist in her recovery. It was these nine words

---

1   Paulo Freire, Pedagogy of the Oppressed. 30th anniversary ed. New York: Continuum, 2000, p. 91.

"there is help available and you can get better" that she heard from her provider and hung on to throughout her recovery. These nine words also resonate in the other nine stories. For Eduardo, Carlos, Estella, and others, having access to a culturally and linguistically responsive program with bilingual and bicultural professionals who understood their cultural and life experiences was what kept giving them hope and see their recovery through.

This book challenges us all regardless of where we come from and live, and whether we are consumers, family members, friends, co-workers, providers, researchers, advocates, policymakers, or administrators. My hope is that this book's content and Pierluigi's poignant personal story along with the other ten stories will give us pause to reflect and contribute to a new day of tolerance, appreciation and celebration in the long quest to understand, treat, and recover from serious mental health conditions among Latino and other underserved populations. Now, fasten your seatbelts and read on...

Sergio Aguilar-Gaxiola, MD, PhD
Professor of Clinical Internal Medicine
Director, Center for Reducing Health Disparities
University of California Davis Health

Insight from my own recovery journey

I am an immigrant and a person in long-term recovery from addiction. I was born in Colombia, South America into an Italian and a Colombian family who ran a pasta and semolina factory that my grandfather and his brother built when they left Italy. I consider myself Colombian by birth, Italian by heritage and American by the grace of God.

I lived in Colombia for 13 years and moved to the United States in 1977 to attend the New York Military Academy located in Cornwall-on-Hudson, New York. I came to the United States to accompany my older brother, Giovanni, who kept getting in trouble at every school he attended, and so my parents felt military school would help him. Gio, as he preferred to be called, was full of life, always involved in several projects and moving very fast; unfortunately his shooting star was unstoppable. Gio passed away young; sometimes I feel he was too big for this world.

In all of my 13 years in Colombia I never saw a drug, not marijuana, not cocaine, not heroin. I did see alcohol since we lived in a very social environment and alcohol was always available. I had my first drink at age 8 at my neighbor's house. It was *Aguardiente*, which translates to 'fire water' similar to what in the U.S. is known as moonshine. I remember feeling happy, throwing up and having another drink. I stumbled my way back home, thankfully we lived next door, and what I remember was that there were no consequences except an *'atta boy'* from my dad when he realized what I had done. My father was a heavy, almost daily drinker who suffered from untreated alcoholism for over 30 years.

But the first time I saw a drug, marijuana, was at the New York Military Academy. One of the members of our troop had some and smoked it during a weekend. I was not interested in it.

In college, I began to see more drugs available but I still was not interested. I drank more than usual and after a year of being there I finally tried cocaine. From the moment I first used it I knew I was hooked.

My addiction lasted three years, from age 19 to 21. During that time I had academic problems and had to withdraw from three universities; I was arrested twice, lost my part time job and alienated my entire family. My recovery date is April 23, 1985.

After my second arrest, which took place in Atlanta, I was so ashamed that I could not call my parents for help. After all I was popular; I was sure that many people would come to my rescue. It was then I found out the hard way that in the drug world there are no friendships, only acquaintances and people who used drugs with you.

When I finally broke down, after 37 days in jail eating corn-based foods three times a day, I called my mother. I had a fantasy that she was going to come and bail me out as she and my dad had done before. But this time was different, she did not.

By this time my father had found his own recovery, and thankfully he remained sober until he passed away. My mother had earned a black belt in Al-Anon and through the strength of their recoveries there was no bailing me out; but there was a lifeline, an offer to go into a substance abuse treatment program.

My public defender negotiated a release to a treatment program in the outskirts of Atlanta but there were no beds available. I was sent to a federal halfway house until a bed opened up at the treatment center. For two weeks I was awakened by an angry albino at 5 a.m. asking for a urine drug test before I began performing the required chores and looking for some part-time work. This was a very scary place and I am grateful my stay there was short.

I was finally released from the halfway house into an inpatient treatment facility where I received individual and group therapy for six weeks. That experience was followed by an outpatient and residential program for six months. I am glad, by the grace of God, I was able to receive a full course of treatment. I entered treatment the last week that I was eligible for benefits under my parents' health insurance. A week later I would have been uninsured and unable to access services.

I did not know what to expect from treatment, I know I was scared and did not want to ruin the rest of my life. Early in my treatment I heard someone say that I shouldn't write down all of the things I wanted to accomplish in recovery, because no matter how long that list was I would have shortchanged myself. And I must admit whoever said it was right. I have received so much in my recovery including things that I would have never had the courage to dream of achieving.

I wanted to lay the groundwork for this book to let you know that this book is extremely personal to me. My family and I have lived the horrors of addiction and mental illness through several generations and seeking and finding cultural and linguistically appropriate treatment in the United States was difficult in the 1980's and it continues to be difficult today.

My father for example, although educated and fluent in English preferred to seek help in Spanish and attended Spanish language support groups. I preferred to receive services in English.

My mother who is also educated and fluent in English also prefers to speak in Spanish when discussing emotional issues. I remember the family therapists that were assigned to me used to struggle when trying to communicate with my mother. The issue was not the language; it was the culture and the lack of cultural understanding by the clinicians. My mother is Colombian, she is well traveled and has lived in several countries. However, her culture is strongly shaped by her Colombian roots. And some of the recovery language the therapists were discussing did not quite meet those cultural expectations. For example words like 'tough love,' or 'co-dependent' did not make sense to my mother at the time and the clinicians struggled to try to explain their meaning. Some of the cultural issues that cause this conflict include our view and understanding of values, attitudes, norms, sociolinguistic factors, socio-political factors, and interactional styles including the ways we think. What is considered a normal close- knit family in Colombia may be interpreted as 'enmeshed' or 'co-dependent' in the United States.

Calling my journey a miracle does not do it justice, I just can't think of a bigger word. From my parents' readiness to send me to treatment, a judge who allowed me the time and the opportunity to get the help I needed to begin my recovery, to the wonderful probation staff, my peers in recovery and my employers who understood recovery was possible and gave me a job in order to remain in Atlanta, to finally receiving a Presidential Pardon from President Clinton, a life changing gesture that opened many doors for me to be able to have a successful life and to be able to give back more than I was given.

I began helping people with behavioral health problems in 1987, after my second recovery anniversary. I did not intend to work in the behavioral health field. I was completing my Bachelor and Master degrees in International Business. But as part of my recovery I began to work in a counseling center and then in an outpatient treatment program and I fell in love with counseling. I returned to school and began a new path. My first fifteen years in recovery were spent working in a residential program for adult clients with addiction and mental illness. The services were delivered in an outpatient setting, but we also offered a residential program because we had many clients who lived outside of Atlanta. During these fifteen years, I had the honor to learn from the best experts in the field at that time, especially Dr. G. Douglas Talbott, who for some reason became interested in me and offered me the support that I could never repay.

During this time, I was able to be part of a team that helped hundreds, possibly thousands, of people achieve recovery. I also witnessed the sadness, destruction and loss of life that this disease brings to those who don't find recovery and to their families. I use the word 'disease' since I was taught and I believe that "the essential feature of a substance use disorder is a cluster of cognitive, behavioral, and physiological symptoms indicating that the individual continues using the substance despite significant substance-related problems" (American Psychiatric Association. (2013). Diagnostic and Statistical Manual of Mental Disorders: DSM-5, p. 483. Washington, D.C: American Psychiatric Association.)

Of all the people who passed through the doors of the organization I first worked at, only one Latino individual was admitted during those fifteen years.

I researched the reasons why that number would be so small and what I found was that although thousands of immigrants from Latin America were moving to Georgia, there were no counseling services available in Spanish anywhere in the state. It reminded me of how difficult it was for my mother, who was bilingual, to fully understand and be able to communicate with clinicians who did not understand the cultural frame from which she was coming. And I pictured how much more difficult getting help must be for all of the individuals with limited English proficiency, and how much they must be suffering.

In 1999 Dr. David Satcher, then the Surgeon General for the United States released "Mental Health: A Report of the Surgeon General (DHHS, 1999)". In this groundbreaking report and its subsequent supplement "Mental Health: Culture, Race and Ethnicity, A Supplement to Mental Health: A Report of the Surgeon General." Dr. Satcher details the barriers that minorities and those with limited English proficiency face when seeking mental health services.

Dr. Satcher stated that "...the organizational barriers include fragmentation of services and lack of availability of services."

He also wrote, "Language, like economic and accessibility differences, can play an important role in why people from other cultures do not seek treatment." And when speaking about what needed to be done, Dr. Satcher encouraged the building of "capacity to provide services in languages other than English." This report was inspirational and it motivated me to do something about the problem.

In 1999 I founded, and for 17 years led, the only Latino clinic in the state of Georgia that was awarded a state license for drug abuse treatment and received national accreditation for behavioral health prevention, intervention and direct clinical services for children, adolescents and adults. The clinic offered services in English, Spanish and Portuguese.

Witnessing the success of the thousands of people my staff and I served is the impetus for writing this book. I want all Latinos, all immigrants and the general public to know that recovery is possible; I want the field of counseling professionals to know that there are evidence-based clinical methods for this population that can help them achieve a better quality of life. And I want government and private agencies to know that they can successfully serve the immigrant population even though immigrants have different levels of acculturation, assimilation as well as different levels of English proficiency.

In this book I present ten stories. The individual's names and other details have been changed for privacy and to protect confidentiality. The vignettes are reconstructed in first-person narratives, consolidating what each client provided during the course of counseling. They highlight their own individual paths to seeking services, what they discovered about themselves and what changes they were able to make in order to improve their lives. I have taken some liberty when reflecting what the individuals said throughout the course of therapy in order to fulfill the narrative. At the end of each chapter I offer practical suggestions that can immediately help those who can identify with that particular story.

All of the individuals featured in this book received culturally responsive services that included cultural and linguistically appropriate services provided by bilingual and bi-cultural clinicians, para-professionals and support staff through a multidisciplinary team. The multidisciplinary team in these cases included bilingual (English/Spanish) Psychiatrist, Psychiatric Physician Assistant, Registered

Nurse, Nutritionist, Psychologist, Licensed Professional Counselors, Licensed Clinical Social Workers, Certified Addiction Counselors, Case Managers, and Recovery Support Service Providers. Services were provided on-site, off-site, in-person, or electronically via telebehavioral health.

I also want to invite you to join me in the international movement to defeat the stigma associated with addiction and mental illness. Recovery is possible, but we must provide services in a way that appeals to the population that needs us the most and has fewer resources. In short, in a way they can access it, when they need it and at a price they can afford.

For clinicians and organizations that want to learn how my team and I were able to achieve so much success with this marginalized population, I will be developing a training program, The Mancini Method ™, which will be available in 2019.

Responding to the needs of immigrants

We are living in an environment where anytime the word *'immigrant'* is mentioned it becomes a polarized conversation. The emotional damage that is being caused to immigrants in the United States by the current administration's public shaming and playing with the future of immigrants for political positioning, is being captured by stories and studies that are documenting the increase in fear, anxiety, depression and other emotional conditions being caused by simply being identified as an immigrant. Children fear their parents won't be at home when they return from school; mothers find themselves unable to perform daily rituals because they feel paralyzed and afraid they will be harassed; children are being bullied at school because they have an ethnic sounding last name, speak with an accent or bring food, traditional to their home country, to eat during lunch. Many immigrants are unwilling to risk their safety in order to meet basic human needs like finding food, clothing and shelter for their family.

It does not have to be this way. The core issues of why many immigrants are suffering in silence are rooted in the fact that most behavioral health providers are unable to adapt to the cultural and linguistic realities taking place in their service areas. In some cases they are willing to adapt and welcome immigrants but they are faced with policy, legislative or other types of barriers that prevent them from providing services.

But as the stories in this book will demonstrate, immigrants are resilient and they can find recovery from mental illness and substance use disorders if they are provided with affordable, culturally and linguistically appropriate services.

In order to successfully help the individuals featured in this book, several factors had to be in place. These factors are a necessity if we are to help the thousands of other individuals with limited English proficiency who are in need of these services. Although these ten stories are from people from Latin America or from the U.S. with Hispanic heritage, these issues affect all persons with Limited English Proficiency regardless of country of origin or ethnic heritage.

Lack or limited access to services is the primary area that needs attention. Access to linguistically appropriate behavioral health and developmental disability services are not proportionally available when compared to the number of individuals reporting their ability to speak English as 'less than very well." In Georgia, for example, there are approximately 500,000 individuals who report that they speak English 'less than very well'. Besides the agency I founded, there are no services in the state to fully serve the immigrant population in the different languages they speak. Title VI of the Civil Rights Act of 1964 defines the denial or delay of medical care due to language barriers as discrimination.

Accessibility also includes other barriers for immigrants and those with limited English proficiency including distrust of the system, misunderstanding of behavioral health care, transportation, childcare, office environment, and office hours to name a few.

Workforce development is another factor that requires policy action. It is well known that we have a shortage of clinicians in general throughout the country and studies show that there are not enough students in clinical programs to replace the aging workforce expected to retire within five years. Today we have entire counties in some states without a single licensed clinician, of any type.

The shortage of clinicians who are bilingual and bi-cultural is even greater.

Solutions for workforce development include changes in policies and even legislative action. The reality is that some states have archaic rules that keep many qualified clinicians from being able to practice where they live simply because they obtained their degrees or practiced somewhere else or their particular school did not require something that is required where they want to practice.

This problem is compounded when looking for bilingual clinicians, including those who serve the deaf and hard of hearing through sign language.

This issue leaves many qualified clinicians who could fill the workforce gaps unable to work and therefore unable to serve many people in need.

The use of interpreters usually is mentioned when discussing linguistic access. But the reality is that interpreters who are trained in behavioral health interpreting vary from state to state. Some states invest in this service and other states don't even have this issue on their radar. When you use interpreters, you are triangulating the clinical process, therefore, training interpreters in behavioral health is critical.

Failure to do so can lead to misunderstanding, misdiagnosing or other problems.

Research normed on the immigrant population is the last factor I will highlight. The issue of culturally responsive evaluation tools and evidence-based-practices (EBPs) is a complicated one, and one that most definitely needs to continue to be discussed in order to bring about change in current practices. One issue that is the fact that evaluation tools are based on standardized questions that were developed for the dominant cultural groups and they include questions that present potential cultural conflicts for a respondent from a different culture. Issues like suicide and sexuality which in some cultures are grounds for punishment or even death.

We must also look at the evidence-based-practices (EBPs) and services that are being used to provide treatment, intervention and prevention services today. Many of them are not developed or normed on the immigrant population but they are still being used either because of not understanding the immigrant population or because the entity funding the services requires that a particular EBP is used regardless of appropriateness for the immigrant or limited English proficient community. Individuals born outside of the United States represent about 14% of the population in the United States. If a researcher cannot find enough members of the immigrant population to include in their research, then they are not looking hard enough or don't want to invest the resources to truly have an exceptional, culturally responsive product.

In creating a program that was culturally and linguistically responsive I was able to set it apart from other agencies. In cultivating and nurturing a multilingual clinical workforce I was able to build a strong team that understood the individuals walking through our doors. It is in knowing and understanding our community and meeting them at their level of need that allowed us to succeed. By the time I stepped down from my agency we were seeing over 100 individuals per day for direct clinical services provided by over 30 bilingual/bi-cultural professionals. We also had bilingual prevention, intervention and recovery services.

The success we have had is solid evidence that affordable, cultural and linguistically appropriate services for immigrants and those with Limited English Proficiency is possible. The Mancini Method ™ will help organizations and clinicians duplicate this success in their own communities.

Chapter One

Carolina's solution to Psychosis and Anxiety

I was going through a tough time, although I tried my very best but I wasn't able to do anything about it and then the worst happened!

I went through an episode of agitation which was later described to me as *"Ataque de Nervios"*, a scary name. I was told that this condition was often compared to panic attacks. My behavior got so out of hand that the police had to be called to restrain me. I was confused, had feelings of terror, my heart was beating so fast that I thought it would jump out of my chest and I was sweating a lot. I was sent to an emergency room where my condition was evaluated and I was referred to another facility to get help.

I am feeling calm today thanks to the treatment I have been going through. Before I got help for my condition I was very anxious and I was under a lot of stress. There was a lot going on in my life, I was emotionally unstable and I was having financial issues.

Most people in this day and age don't believe in black magic but I do, and I also believe that every problem that I have been facing including the episode that I had was due to a curse that was placed on me. In my family this is very common. Even people who go to church still sometimes go and see the *'brujo'* (witch doctor) to have curses removed or to try to find out what is going to happen in the near future.

I am from Nicaragua and I am an immigrant in the United States.

Like many immigrants in this country my social and emotional support network is very small. I have probably lived more than my fair share of life and I say that because I have seen more financial stress, more agitation, more emotional stress, more sadness and more anger than most of the people by the age of 43.

I started working harder than ever before after my husband was deported and I was left all alone with my two children although due to all these hardships I was able to bring a lot of positive changes in my life.

My husband Ramiro used to beat me up, he would get physically aggressive, he would get jealous for whatever reason and often he would not allow me to leave the house. He was very possessive and thought that when I went out all the men would look at me and he did not like that. I have friends who also go through the same thing. He felt that if he did not control me he was not a real man. He did not give me any money for daily expenses and he did not allow me to work, everyone has their limits and I was way past mine.

This was not the only physical abuse I had experienced in my life. I had reached the end of my rope but it was not an easy decision to call the police. You see, the abuse by my husband was not a unique event; it was the last in series of abuses I had experienced. At work, I struggled with a boss who threatened me, made unwelcomed advances toward me, and made my years at this job a living hell. Through all this, I kept my mouth shut. I can just hear my mother saying: *"¡No te quejes tanto! No eres la única a lo que eso le pasa. Esto es parte de nuestra vida. Yo he sufrido por lo mismo."* (Don't complain so much! You are not the only one who goes through this. This is part of our lives. I have also suffered like that.) Violence had become so normal that it didn't even bother me when I was shot.

I called the police again and told them all about my husband's abuse and this time they helped me, but not in the way I was expecting. My husband was arrested and was placed under a deportation order, and soon after that he was deported. I never expected that Ramiro would be placed on a deportation order. I wanted the police to intervene to stop him from abusing me but I did not want them to do something that would bring such devastation to my children and me. You see, having a possessive and over controlling husband also meant that I depended on him for money and was not used to making it on my own.

At first, I was afraid of what would become of my children and me, but with time I made my peace with it, after a long and hard struggle I was finally able to provide for my children.

My life hasn't been easy, I was raped at the age of 17 and I had to go through an abortion because of it. It was not easy but then when is it easy? I was molested by an uncle at the age of 12 and it had an everlasting impact on my life. As a result of all these things I was emotionally traumatized for a long time. Somehow I was strong enough to never contemplate suicide.

I am the first person in my family to openly admit and seek help for my mental illness. None of my family members have ever admitted an addiction to either drugs or alcohol and no one had ever shown signs of mental illness – at least they never admitted it publicly. In Nicaragua, families just keep their problems hidden because it brings shame to a family to expose something like mental illness. Mental illness tends to be seen as a reflection of something the family did, something bad for which now we are being punished. Addiction is seen as a weakness of character, not as a disease. Then there's our religion and our belief that you don't burden others with your problems because it's selfish. You bear your crosses silently.

I value myself as a law-abiding person and besides traffic tickets I have not had any problems with the police. I get along with my children and with my friends, I have never physically punished my children or have become violent with any of my friends. One area where I know that I want to improve is my education, I was never able to get a formal education, but now I enrolled in a class to help me learn how to read and write in English, something I am very proud of.

Every coin has two sides and my life is no exception, just as there is a dark side to my life there is also the one filled with light and hope, I have seen good times too.

But I am often filled with anxiety and fear, fear of what is ahead of me.

When I showed up at the facility to begin treatment, I was friendly and cooperative with the person helping me with my admission process. I was very nervous. I didn't know what I should say and how much I should say. I worried about what they might think of me, of making a bad impression, of coming across like an ignorant *campensina* (peasant). I didn't pour out all my problems because I didn't want to come across too self-centered and I also didn't want to expose myself too much to someone I didn't know or trust. I was told after my evaluation that I minimized the problems I was having and sometimes I make rash decisions. I became aware and embarrassed when I realized that for this appointment I did not dress well and I appeared disheveled. But after a while I was able to feel more comfortable and share the things that were causing me so much anxiety and fear.

I was told that I have general anxiety and that some of the symptoms I had like feeling hot, having extreme palpitation, shortness of breath and feeling like I might faint anytime were all part of my illness. This information helped me but it also scared me because I did not know if I was going to die from this.

I was also diagnosed with a psychotic disorder, panic attacks, depression and sexual trauma. All of these words scared me even more and I asked myself where did I get all of these problems? Did I cause them? Did someone give them to me? My counselor was very gentle when she explained what those words meant. She explained that a diagnosis for mental illness is just like any other illness, for example, if I go to the doctor and he tells me that I have a cold.

I was not given many answers the first day but I was told that there was help available and I could get better. I liked that; it was reassuring.

I was told that the counselors were Latino and they spoke English and Spanish and that I would be assigned one main counselor but that there was a team of professionals that would be working with me. I did not understand much so I hung on to the words I heard earlier "there is help available, and you can get better."

At the beginning of my treatment I was given individual therapy with a very nice lady and medication for anxiety, I was also told that I would be attending the women's trauma group, that I would have another counselor help me with something called recovery support and that I would see the psychiatrist to help manage my medication and see if there was anything else I needed to work on.

I did not know much about medication but a very nice nurse sat down with me and explained to me what the medicines they were recommending do, how long they would take to work and how they would make me feel. This helped a lot since I didn't like taking medications.

One of the greatest gifts I found was that since I couldn't communicate properly in English at that time all my treatments were delivered in Spanish by Spanish speaking counselors.

They said that they would be able to help me with my anxiety which included feelings of desperation and sadness, isolation, low self-esteem, and the stress from the trauma I suffered as a result of domestic violence.

I had a wonderful treatment team. They were open and friendly and during every session they made sure I was comfortable and felt safe to talk about anything. I received support, encouragement and love. The counselors did their best to help me by using the different ways to help me which they called 'interventions'. They identified the negative thoughts and behaviors that contributed to my stress and helped me learn new skills, like relaxation, so that I would be able to face challenges and reduce my anxiety.

This was all new to me. In my country it's very difficult to find counselors. Where I lived we did not have telephones or internet nor did we talk about getting help for our mental health. I would have gone to a healer to have these curses removed from me. But here, these counselors took baby steps to help me see that there were other ways to get better and if I trusted them I could learn those ways. I had nothing to lose so I decided to trust them.

The counselors taught me how to do new things that they called 'strategies' which included how to stop my thoughts before they went too far, positive affirmations, meditation, relaxation, and decision-making skills to help me learn to cope with my anxiety, sadness, and feelings of hopelessness. I believe all those things had a positive effect because I began to feel better.

They helped me understand things that I did not understand and some of the behaviors that contributed to my co-dependency. Like when I put the feelings of others before my own feelings.

They helped me recognize that I had values, talents, assets, and qualities that could help me think better off and respect myself. I had never thought of these when I was growing up. I was not used to thinking about looking at the strengths I already had in me. It just wasn't something that I had been brought up to think about to help me cope with life.

I was taught how to use deep breathing and something new called mindfulness on a daily basis especially whenever I was worried, and I was able to identify two or three triggers of my constant concerns that increased my heart palpitations. Some of these things at first seemed strange: deep breathing and mindfulness. These were new to me but the counselor encouraged me to try them out. I trusted my counselor; she was Latina like me and if she believed in these things I felt I could, too.

Today I have a new relationship with a wonderful man. My counselors helped me learn how to express my feelings to my partner daily so that I might be able to have a healthy romantic relationship. I also learned how to have a better relationship with my children.

After six months of counseling I completed my treatment and I feel it was successful. It was hard but I kept moving forward. Now after six months of having completed my treatment I continue to manage my anxiety a lot better, I feel better, I communicate better and I work daily on my recovery.

I realized that I was given a wonderful opportunity and I committed to continue practicing my new skills, to see the doctor as I needed and to stay in touch with my counselors.

IMMEDIATE SUGGESTIONS FOR PEOPLE WHO IDENTIFY WITH SOME PARTS OF CAROLINA'S STORY

Disclaimer: Mental health and addiction issues should not be addressed alone. Please seek professional help to reach the highest level of emotional well-being possible. These suggestions can be used as support for professional help or for people who are not suffering as seriously as Carolina.

1. Deep Breathing Technique - The 4-7-8 Exercise

The 4-7-8 breathing exercise is very simple, it can be done anywhere, and you can do it at any time. The 4-7-8 breathing technique, championed by practitioner and teacher of integrative medicine Andrew Weill, is simple and worth trying. It's free, quick and doesn't require equipment. Before you begin, sit with your back straight and place the tip of your tongue on the roof of your mouth just above your teeth and keep it there throughout the exercise.

- Exhale completely through your mouth - quite forcefully so you make a "whoosh" sound.
- Close your mouth and inhale quietly and softly through your nose for a mental count of **four.**
- Hold your breath and count to **seven.**
- Exhale completely through your mouth, making another whoosh sound for **eight** seconds in one large breath.
- Inhale again and repeat the cycle three times for a total of four breaths.

Remember: All inhaling breaths must be quiet and through your nose and all exhaling breaths must be loud and through your mouth.

2. Positive Affirmations: Positive affirmations are directly related to the chemistry of our brain, so repeating them several times, can manifest a change in how we think and how we behave. The power of positive affirmations lies in their ability to improve our emotional state.

Positive affirmations should have three basic elements:

1. Be written in the first person, using present tense and using a positive / affirmative language.
2. They must have an emotional effect.
3. They must be true for you.

For example, in the case of Carolina, a positive affirmation may be: "I am going to attract healthy people into my life."

Chapter 2

Eduardo's solution to Alcoholism, Panic and Anxiety

My name is Eduardo, I am 30 years old and I was born in Guatemala. I've been living in the United States for four years and I asked for help after ending up in a hospital due to excessive drinking during a holiday celebration. I used to drink an average of 18 beers every time I drank 4-5 times per week. I began to drink at the age of 20, and I would drink to get drunk and for no other reason. I think the main reason for my heavy drinking was a feeling of panic that overwhelmed me completely until I would begin to drink. Alcohol seemed to calm me. I noticed an increase in panic attacks and heavy drinking over the past three years after my father passed away. There was also something that was out of the ordinary, whenever I had a panic attack, I felt like urinating and the feeling was like someone was grabbing my private parts.

When I arrived for treatment, I reported pain in my chest, and near my heart, my right arm would fall asleep, I felt some numbing on my face, and my hands would get cold at times. After a complete medical examination, the tests on my heart and all follow up tests were all normal.

I was inappropriately touched by a male family friend several times when I was 12 years old. Whenever I remembered this abuse, I felt panic attacks, and I would numb that feeling with alcohol. I would get angry whenever I thought about the abuse, but instead of telling anyone or hurting anyone, I would just get drunk. I never thought about suicide; I guess drinking was slowly killing me.

I used to consider myself a heterosexual but due to the abuse and the memories I would often lose interest in all sex. After drinking in excess, I had hangovers, blackouts, withdrawal symptoms, and I could not sleep very well. I have a sister who suffered from depression and my father suffered from alcoholism. Besides these problems with alcohol I have never had any medical problems, surgeries or hospitalizations.

I started to feel guilty about my drinking; I think that when I began treatment I was feeling depressed. I believe that my drinking caused problems in my relationships with family and friends. Over the past four months, before getting help, I began to isolate myself, began to miss work a lot and for several days at a time I would not even leave my house.

Alcohol was my only drug. I tried cocaine and marijuana a couple of times but didn't like how they made me feel.

I usually work as a cook. I never finished school; my education stopped in the sixth grade while I was living in Guatemala. I dropped out of school to work and help my family.

When I started counseling I was full of anxiety, fear and apprehension. I would be polite but felt I did not have a lot of energy to relate to people. I was very aware of my problems except for the times when I could not remember recent events or had thoughts that were confusing. In Guatemala the government created clinics with psychologists so people could get help, but I never thought I had a problem.

In my family, we were always taught to be polite and dress well, with clean clothes. To respect others and to sit up straight. That's exactly how I showed up for my appointments, well dressed, soft spoken and with good posture.

I was feeling hopeless worthless and helpless; I had times when I felt very happy, very talkative, impulsively spending money, I had a lot of energy and little need for sleep for up to three days at a time. For all the time I was awake, I did not have any beliefs out of the ordinary nor saw or heard anything unusual. I was told later that this was called having periods of mania.

My counselors told me I had something called alcohol dependence, anxiety, agoraphobia (fear of and avoidance of places or situations that might cause you to panic) and panic disorder.

I began to receive individual therapy with a wonderful therapist; the doctor gave me medication for anxiety and panic disorder and I began to attend a group counseling with other people having problems with alcohol. Since I speak, read and understand Spanish better than English all my services were provided in Spanish.

In the group, I learned that getting better was going to take a lot of time and effort. I needed to learn how to stop drinking, how to be around people again and how to begin overcoming my periods of panic.

My counselors began working with me in identifying the things that stressed me out every day (e.g., work, social, family relationships). I was taught new techniques to build social and personal skills to manage everyday challenges, stressors and emotions.

In the group sessions, I realized the harm that alcohol had been doing to my body, I was provided with medication and new tools to identify the triggers that pushed me to drink so heavily.

The first step was not to drink alcohol, one minute at a time sometimes, then, to manage common day-to-day challenges and to build confidence in maintaining them without alcohol or any other drugs.

I began to learn how to engage in social and recreational activities with my girlfriend. I began with one activity per week for three months to start and most of the activities should be outside of the home.

After five months of counseling and support I realized that I was feeling much better. I was no longer experiencing depressed mood, panic attacks or alcohol cravings. I am continuing to go out into social situations with my girlfriend and I am also going to church where I am receiving a lot of support. I plan to continue taking my medications as prescribed and follow up with the psychiatrist as recommended.

I am happy to say that I now have a stable social life with family, friends; a girlfriend who cares about me and many new friends at church. I am sleeping better and have not had a drink since I entered treatment.

IMMEDIATE SUGGESTIONS FOR PEOPLE WHO IDENTIFY WITH SOME PARTS OF EDUARDO'S STORY

Disclaimer: Mental health and addiction issues should not be addressed alone. Please seek professional help to reach the highest level of emotional well-being possible. These suggestions can be used as support for professional help or for people who are not suffering as seriously as Eduardo.

1. **Recovery Support Meetings** - Merriam-Webster Dictionary defines support groups as a group of people with common experiences and concerns who provide emotional and moral support for one another. https://www.merriam-webster.com/dictionary/supportgroup. For alcohol, drugs or other addictions there are plenty of support groups and someone who wants to recover from any of these illnesses will need the support of others who have been through it. For a comprehensive list of Self-Help, Peer Support, and Consumer Groups - Self-Help Groups (Addiction) visit https://findtreatment.samhsa.gov/locator/link-focSelfGP

2. **Setting boundaries** – A boundary is a rule, a guide that you can create to let other people know what behavior is acceptable to you so they know how you would expect them to behave. For example, for Eduardo, a boundary may be to let other people know that he is recovering from alcoholism and being near alcohol may cause a relapse, therefore he prefers if others don't drink around him. To set your own boundaries you must look within yourself and find out what is important to you, why you would set that boundary and what you are willing to do if someone chooses to violate the boundary you have set.

Chapter 3

Carlos' solution for Impulse Control and Marijuana

My son Carlos is a 13-year-old teenager with a history of behavioral problems both at school and at home that have been escalating over the past year. He is currently enrolled in school in Norcross, Georgia where he was born and is attending the 7th grade. My son also started smoking Marijuana. He started having problems at the age of 10. He started being interested in girls and wanted a girlfriend and as days went by he was becoming more and more irritable and bad tempered. He was taken to a psychologist to learn about sex education and to attend to the anger issues he was having. He was seen twice a month for about one year. We also had some family therapy, in the hope that it might make things better.

After he began to date, he became more disrespectful at home and at school. He was suspended from school 8 times in the last 12 months. The school system was ready to transfer him to an alternative school if his behavior had continued to be disruptive at school. At home, he has lost all his privileges including the use of his cell phone or any other electronic devices including the computer and any video games. He was disrespectful to me and called me a bitch often. He would always say that he feels bored and angry and that he doesn't have anything to help him deal with his stress.

He said he feels "stressed" at school and was having trouble academically, and that he used Marijuana only to relax.

During his evaluation, he told the counselor that he is "popular" at school. He shared the fact proudly; he was also proud of being social and having a girlfriend that was one year behind him at school. One of the times he got in trouble at school was for kissing at school. Other reasons for his suspensions were being disruptive, fighting, being disrespectful to teachers and arguing. Academically my son was failing nearly all of his classes.

During his first session at the clinic, Carlos was uninterested, he was cooperative but it was like pulling teeth. He seemed like he did not trust anyone. My son was diagnosed with Disruptive Behavior Disorder, Cannabis abuse and Parent-Child Relational Problem.

My son receives individual therapy, group therapy, recovery support services and random drug tests. It was also recommended that he see the psychiatrist for medication evaluation.

The major problems that need treatment were the disruptive behavior and the marijuana use. The counselors helped him look at ways that would help him decrease or stop the use of marijuana. They helped him identify and utilize new, drug-free, social activities and helped him see the benefits of being involved in these activities.

Carlos also began to use the tutoring service the clinic had for its adolescents to help him improve his grades. Carlos liked this because he began to see results right away. He participated in discussions and activities around living a drug-free life.

I learned how to validate my son's feelings, no matter what they were, they were his feelings and I needed to learn how to respect that. The counselor told me that feelings are feelings, they are not good or bad. They are different from behaviors; I don't have to accept or validate negative or unhealthy behaviors.

In time, my son was able to improve grades for all classes. He was able to identify ways in which drinking and smoking marijuana has negatively affected him and his school work. He learned coping strategies (playing sports, calling a friend for support, listening to music) to prevent him from smoking marijuana or using alcohol. He made supportive friends who did not influence him to use substances. He also started having dinner with me instead of isolating himself.

After four months, he stated that he had decreased his marijuana use; had learned the consequences of continued use; had improved his grades and was learning how to better communicate with me. His behavior has improved, and his grades have also improved.

Carlos has not had any further behavior problems at school. I am still concerned that he did not completely stopped using marijuana. But as the counselor reminds me, this is about progress, not perfection.

IMMEDIATE SUGGESTIONS FOR PEOPLE WHO IDENTIFY WITH SOME PARTS OF CARLOS' STORY

Disclaimer: Mental health and addiction issues should not be addressed alone. Please seek professional help to reach the highest level of emotional well-being possible. These suggestions can be used as support for professional help or for people who are not suffering as seriously as Carlos.

1. **Tutoring** – This service is one of the most beneficial services to help youth who are experimenting with alcohol, drugs and other risky behaviors and who are having academic difficulty. Often young people will use alcohol and drugs because they are bored. But many times that translates to "I don't know how to study and am doing poorly I school, therefore I will use alcohol and drugs." But, in my experience, once we empower them academically, they soar and the risky behaviors tend to rapidly decrease and even stop. There are many types of tutoring, peer tutors (by other students), professional tutors, in-home tutors, on-line tutors, and others. Tutoring is helping students improve their learning strategies in order to promote independence and empowerment. The purpose of tutoring is to help students help themselves, assisting them to become independent learners and thus no longer needing a tutor.
2. **Involve children in meal planning** – One of the easiest ways to guarantee that children want to have dinner with the entire family is to involve them in all aspects of meal preparation. Begin by visiting https://www.choosemyplate.gov/ to get all the information you need. My Plate is a free program that will help the entire family find your healthy eating style and build it throughout your lifetime. Everything you eat and drink matters. The right mix can help you be healthier now and in the future. Here are some tips to involve everyone: 1) find out their favorite meals and take turns making one person's favorite dish each night; 2) sit down together and write down the ingredients you will need; 3) review grocery store ads; 4) clip coupons together; 5) ask the children to participate in meal preparation and cooking; and 6) set the table together.

3. **Parents - Seek Professional Help:** Helping an adolescent who is struggling with substance abuse and/or a mental health issue is not easy. The mental health of the entire family is affected when one member is having difficulties, especially if that member is a child. Mental health is very valuable and we should not deny ourselves and our families the gift of being happy and being able to function fully in our lives with everything we want to do. To find help, you can go to https://findtreatment.samhsa.gov/

Chapter 4

Estella's solution to Bipolar Disorder and Anxiety Solution

I felt depressed every day, anxious all night, and I wasn't able to sleep. I felt very tired all the time.

I had trouble concentrating and I cried often. I felt guilty about everything that had gone wrong in my life and always blamed myself for things even when I knew it was not my fault at all. I had periods of anxiety especially whenever I found myself in small enclosed places including the bathroom, which I would always use with the door open because I felt anxious otherwise. Whenever I felt anxious I used a different method to deal with it, whatever would be most effective at the time. Sometimes I would eat large quantities of food to comfort me and sometimes I would eat sweets. Hopelessness was all that I felt. Physical, sexual and emotional trauma were part of my daily routine during an abusive marriage for a period of 10 years.

I'm a 40-year-old woman born in New York but I lived in Colombia most of my life. I first started to seek help due to my depression and anxiety. I had many depressive episodes in the past but this one was worse than all the ones before. I had been feeling very depressed and fatigued for about three weeks. I had little desire to do anything and I was crying a lot. It had been a while since I was interested in activities that I once used to enjoy. My lack of desire and interest had been going for the past six months. A week before I sought help I had a fleeting thought about crashing into the back of a car but stopped myself because my daughter was with me. This incident was the final trigger that pushed me to seek help for my situation. I have no suicidal plans or any intent to hurt myself but I admit that I sometimes used to think that death was the best option.

I now live in a house with my boyfriend and my children. Like I wrote before I was born in New York but was taken to Colombia at an early age. I along with my 3 other siblings were raised by both of my parents. During the time that I spent with my family I always felt that my mother never accepted me. I also don't remember my childhood very well but something that do remember vividly is that I was always wondering why I looked different from my siblings and thus why I always felt left out. On the other hand, I had a very good close relationship with my father growing up.

As time passed things changed, I now have a close relationship with both of my parents, I'm happy it turned out this way. I have very few friends here in the states and one thing that always saddens me is that I don't get to see my friends in Colombia very much.

I completed my formal education and graduated high school, college and post-graduate studies in medicine. I had a medical practice license in Colombia, but I wasn't able to practice medicine in the United States due to the difficulty in transferring medical and/or clinical licenses here from abroad. The closest I can get to practicing here is by working as a medical assistant.

I am usually a straight shooter, tell-it-like-it-is type of person, I think that is usually best. So, when I was being diagnosed I asked the clinician to be straight with me. I was told that I have been diagnosed with Bipolar II Disorder, also known as Manic Depression where sometimes I feel extremely happy and other times extremely sad. I was familiar with the diagnosis and the symptoms.

In Colombia I never thought about getting help. The stigma associated with mental illness was too much to bear, so I decided not to get help while I was there.

Things here were different. I felt comfortable in the place that I found. They had people who spoke Spanish and made me feel welcomed. Even though I did not do a psychiatric rotation I was familiar with behavioral health and struggled with being teachable now that I was the client and not the doctor.

I followed their advice, and I began individual therapy, a support group and saw the psychiatrist who placed me on medication to help me get better. The psychiatrist was familiar with the struggles I may be having by sitting on the other side of the desk but he made me feel comfortable and I felt respected. This made it easier for me to follow his recommendations.

Although I am fluent in English I have always felt more comfortable speaking about my emotions in Spanish. Therefore, I requested that my treatment be delivered in Spanish.

Identifying the things that caused me to experience depression and anxiety was a key part of my treatment. The staff helped me learn new healthy coping skills to deal with my symptoms of depression and anxiety. I also learned other skills which helped me a lot. One other thing that was given a lot of importance during my treatment was to learn how to establish boundaries with my children.

Now after six months, I have no symptoms of depression or hypomania and I was able to accomplish all of my treatment goals. I was able to participate in self-care activities. I successfully identified triggers for my feelings of depression and anxiety and have acquired and practiced healthy coping skills. I was also able to establish and keep boundaries with my children and my relationship with them has improved a lot. I can see the improvement and I can see my self-esteem increase since the beginning of treatment.

IMMEDIATE SUGGESTIONS FOR PEOPLE WHO IDENTIFY WITH SOME PARTS OF ESTELLA'S STORY

Disclaimer: Mental health and addiction issues should not be addressed alone. Please seek professional help to reach the highest level of emotional well-being possible. These suggestions can be used as support for professional help or for people who are not suffering as seriously as Estella's.

1. **Exercise** – Many studies confirm what we have heard for many years. Exercise is essential, it benefits our physical and emotional needs to have a healthy, active life. But for so many of us, especially if we are suffering from depression, getting started is very difficult. These five steps on how to get started are from Live Science.
   a. **Be Safe** – Safety first. You should never begin an exercise program before checking with your doctor. If you have a health condition, speak with your doctor about whether you'll need to take any precautions when you exercise.
   b. **Enjoy yourself** – Pick an exercise that you enjoy doing. This could be a more traditional form of exercise, like jogging or going to the gym; sports like tennis or soccer; or even a dance class.
   c. **Start Gradually** – Start out with a fairly light activity, and gradually increase the duration and intensity of exercise. The goal is to complete 30 minutes of exercise a day, five days a week. These 30 minutes can be done all at once, or broken up into 10-minute increments.
   d. **Don't Overdo it** – Avoid high-impact exercises, which involve lots of jumping or ballistic movements, because these can lead to injury when you are first starting out.
   e. **Set goals** – Set goals to keep yourself motivated in your exercise, like running a 5K or improving your time. You might also consider getting a friend to exercise with you to hold you accountable.
2. **Setting Limits with your Children** – There are several schools of thoughts that address how to set limits with your children. The truth is that every family and every situation is different.

You must be honest with yourself regarding your ability to enforce or keep a limit once it has been set. One of the problems many parents have is that they set limits but when it's broken they do not enforce a consequence. This teaches the child that limits and boundaries must not apply to them because there are no consequences if they are broken. Therefore choose limits that are age appropriate, that are clear and that, if broken, you will be able to enforce the consequence. For example, one popular limit is limiting 'screen time' for children. So if you want to limit your children to two hours of video or computer games per day you must:

   a. **Communicate the reason for the limit clearly** – because it can affect their ability to sleep
   b. **Communicate the consequence if the limit is broken** – They will lose the video games for two days
   c. **Be able to live with yourself when you impose the consequence.**

3. **Deep Breathing Technique** - The 4-7-8 Exercise

The 4-7-8 breathing exercise is very simple, it can be done anywhere, and you can do it at any time. The 4-7-8 breathing technique, championed by practitioner and teacher of integrative medicine Andrew Weill, is simple and worth trying. It's free, quick and doesn't require equipment.

Before you begin, sit with your back straight and place the tip of your tongue on the roof of your mouth just above your teeth and keep it there throughout the exercise.

- Exhale completely through your mouth - quite forcefully so you make a "whoosh" sound.
- Close your mouth and inhale quietly and softly through your nose for a mental count of four.
- Hold your breath and count to seven.
- Exhale completely through your mouth, making another whoosh sound for eight seconds in one large breath.
- Inhale again and repeat the cycle three times for a total of four breaths.

Remember: All inhaling breaths must be quiet and through your nose and all exhaling breaths must be loud and through your mouth.

Chapter 5

Rosa's solution to Obsession and Depression Solutions

My name is Rosa, I was born in Honduras, I'm 36 years old and I came to the United States thirteen years ago at the age of 23 along with my 4-year-old son at the time. I had a history of suffering from Obsessive Compulsive Disorder (OCD) and received counseling and medication ten years ago for about two years. At the time, I was placed on Prozac for two months but I didn't like some of the side effects of the medication. I received counseling five years ago, and the focus of the therapy at that time was the separation from my husband and symptoms of depression. I sought help once again because of a relapse in my symptoms of OCD and some depression symptoms like suddenly crying, low energy, low self-esteem and some anxiety.

The OCD symptoms that resurfaced included checking the stove up to three times every time I left the house and checking the house alarm or the front door lock three times each time before leaving the house. I started to have bad thoughts that started bothering me a lot such as "something bad is going to happen to my son or to me." If I tried to stop myself from engaging in my obsessive rituals I felt a lot of anxiety and I wasn't able to concentrate. If I ever left my house without doing my rituals I would feel anxious all day long until I got back home and performed those rituals. I also started to kneel and started asking God for help more and more.

A week before I went to seek help I was more depressed than ever. Part of that feeling came from recently being intimate with my ex-husband. I criticized myself and constantly made myself believe that I was trash and not worth anything. I wasn't able to stop beating myself up for what I did. I was shaming myself for returning to counseling after a long period of absence from those symptoms.

My son is now 17 years old and I run my own business, I can provide for myself and my family. When my OCD symptoms returned, I didn't socialize often, my best friend moved out of state, and I didn't have a lot of other friends at that time. My son and I took a short vacation, but we haven't done anything else since.

Although my father, my uncles and my ex-husband drink heavily I never had a taste for alcohol, and I don't like being around people who drink excessively. I get along with my mother who lives close to me; we talk to each other often. I believe one of my brothers also suffers from OCD but has not been diagnosed. He is much stronger than me and deals with his problem very well. One of my sisters also suffers from depression.

I am a pretty healthy person. The only medical problem I ever had was a fall when I was a little girl. I hit my head and to this day I suffer from summer, seasonal, migraine headaches.

I sought help because I felt anxiety, fear and apprehension. I was glad to find help in Spanish. Everyone at the clinic was friendly and helpful. I am a friendly person naturally and was very comfortable telling my story, after all I was here to get help.

When all the questions stopped, the staff confirmed what I had shared earlier, that I showed symptoms that meet the diagnosis for obsessive-compulsive disorder and Depressive Disorder. I was assigned a counselor to have individual therapy with and a psychiatrist to evaluate medications that can also help me get better.

I was very glad that I found this agency and that they knew how to help me. In Honduras, there are some places that provide help but only if you are lucky enough to live in a few areas that have them.

To help me overcome the obsessive-compulsive disorder symptoms I started slowly. I began checking the stove and front door of my house only before leaving. I would journal exactly what I did so I can share it with my counselor. Slowly I began to feel an increase in my sense of self-control and feelings. I learned how to keep a worry journal and use the information to identify sources of anxiety, normalize feelings, and dispute distorted thoughts. This activity helped me a lot in pinpointing the areas where I needed improvement.

I learned acceptance, which was fairly hard for me but in the end, I did it. I learned new skills to manage my anxiety. Through experiential exercises I learned how to experience and practice new skills. I was given the opportunity to use relaxation techniques such as breathing. I also learned how to develop positive counter thoughts, which is when you think a negative thought about your health, you can then counter that negative thought by making a new thought that is positive and about good health.

Now after five months, I feel excellent. I have been able to decrease my obsessive behaviors, and some days I don't even have to check the door anymore. I was able to meet all of my personal goals, and I am working and providing for my family. I was able to let go of the relationship with my ex-husband that was unhealthy. I have built a supportive community around me and I'm focused on my future goals. I feel confident with my skills and look forward to a healthier future.

IMMEDIATE SUGGESTIONS FOR PEOPLE WHO IDENTIFY WITH SOME PARTS OF ROSA'S STORY

Disclaimer: Mental health and addiction issues should not be addressed alone. Please seek professional help to reach the highest level of emotional well-being possible. These suggestions can be used as support for professional help or for people who are not suffering as seriously as Rosa.

1. **Keep a 'Worry Journal'** – this technique is widely utilized by people with and without a mental health issue. There is a lot of power in writing down your worries. It unlocks the fear we associate with it and it allows us to come up with clarifications and a plan to defuse them.
   a. **Choose your type of journal.** Pen and paper or electronic methods work the same. Your just have to use it.
   b. **Write down the issues and/or behaviors that cause the worry.** This could be things like being late, the health condition of a family member, and a fear of something bad happening. In Rosa's case, we can use the repeated action of checking the lock. So you would write "I check the lock three times before I leave the house."
   c. **Clarify the fear.** Once you identify it, you need to clarify it. For example, is Rosa's fear that the lock would not work and therefore someone could get in? In your journal, you would write exactly that, "I am afraid that the lock won't work and someone can break into my place."
   d. **Defuse the fear.** This is easier said than done and it may take more than one try so don't worry. Here you would write the ways you can find comfort that the lock will work once you locked it the first time. For example, "I just bought this lock and it's one of the strongest in the market", "After I lock the door I turn the handle and it does not open", and "My friend also tried to open the door after I locked it and she could not get in".

2. **Muscle Relaxation** – There are several techniques for muscle relaxation that can help release anxiety and alleviate depression. Muscle Relaxation teaches you how to relax your muscles through a two-step process. First, you systematically tense muscle groups in your body, such as your neck and shoulders. Next, you release the tension and notice how your muscles feel when you relax them. This exercise will help you to lower your overall tension and stress levels, and help you relax when you are feeling anxious. It can also help reduce physical problems such as stomachaches and headaches, as well as improve your sleep.

Chapter Six

Ofelia's solution to Anxiety and Mood Disorders

I've always been a nervous person. My anxiety took a turn for the worse and increased two years ago, after my aunt and uncle passed away. I started to have more stress, different physical complaints, menstrual irregularities, headaches and dizziness. I went to different doctors and they reassured me that it was just stress due to my aunt and uncle passing away.

I am a 28-year-old woman from Oaxaca, Mexico and I've been having anxiety since I was 13 years old. The first time I was diagnosed with it was when I was 16. At the age of 13, I was diagnosed with arrhythmia but no treatment was needed and none was recommended by the doctors. A week before I sought help, I had my first full panic attack, and was taken to the hospital. I felt palpitations, fear, dizziness, pressure in my ears, stiffness in my neck and fear of breathing. I was afraid of dying and I was also afraid that something bad was going to happen to me.

Another factor that forced me to get help was a health news segment about the heart, I felt very afraid and had a panic attack there and then. It was so severe that I ended up in the emergency room, I was checked, had an EKG and cardiac work up done and everything came back normal. I was diagnosed with a fast heartbeat, palpitations, and a urinary tract infection at that time.

During my checkup at the hospital I was referred to a psychiatrist. I was feeling anxious ever since I went to the hospital, worried about my health and something happening to me, feeling nauseous, having diarrhea, shaking, feeling pressure in my head, and shortness of breath. I have insomnia, at that time I was sleeping for about six hours, waking up every couple of hours. Television news, in general triggered more anxiety and I admit worrying about everything, and it's been this way for the last two years. I worry about bad things happening to my kids.

I had to quit my job because I felt very stressed out and didn't have control over the things that happened there. Two years ago, I ended an extra marital affair that lasted eight months, and I felt very guilty about it. I've never had any homicidal or suicidal ideation, but I have punched myself twice, hard, out of frustration. But then, isn't human nature that when you can't do anything to change or affect anything that matters to you the only way is to hurt your own self? Just like people going on hunger strikes, it only hurts them, yet they do it because they feel it's the only thing they can control.

I was born in Mexico and raised by my parents with my younger sister. My father was very controlling and jealous of my mother, he did not demonstrate any affection to my sister and me, and I was afraid of him for being verbally abusive. My parents argued a lot. Dad was emotionally abusive towards my mom and me. My mother left for the United States when I was 18 years old and I was heartbroken and suffered a lot with the separation. I moved in with a boyfriend but separated two years later.

The days after I went to the ER, it was very difficult to function, and I was feeling hopeless and helpless. I felt depressed. My appetite decreased, and I experienced lack of energy and motivation.

I suffered post-partum depression after my son was born. As a teenager, I had anger problems due to having to hide my emotions in front of my parents. I also had sleep problems, I went to see a doctor once and was prescribed Valerian Root to help me sleep which helped a little.

I have had periods of elevated mood, increased energy, racing thoughts, decreased need for sleep which would often last for days, mood swings over the last two years including impulsive decisions.

At the age of 20 I came to the United States. Three months after getting to the US I started a relationship with the father of my children and we are still together. My husband doesn't know about the affair I had two years ago.

I was very anxious when I went to ask for help. But I was honest and did not hold back. I really wanted help, and I figured that if I don't tell them what's bothering me, then I am just wasting everyone's time.

I was told I had anxiety and that they could help me, that I was not alone and that I would meet others who had been through what I was going thorough and they got better.

I received individual therapy, group therapy and recovery support services by wonderful people. I also saw the psychiatrist for medication to help me get better.

From the beginning my counselor wanted me to focus on my anxiety, the fear of having panic attacks and my lack of motivation for exercise. She helped me identify the reasons why I felt anxious and taught me new skills to manage my anxiety. The skills to cope with anxiety was something that helped me a lot more than I initially expected. I was also able to identify the barriers interfering with job search and placement.

I identified personal values, talents, assets and qualities in order to instill self-confidence and motivation. I could identify and overcome triggers for anxiety symptoms like palpations. I acquired relaxation skills and motivational skills that helped me a lot.

I can see how much I have improved; there has been a significant reduction in my anxiety. Going out alone is not a problem anymore I am neither afraid nor anxious. I have learned the ability to manage my anxiety. I was able to secure a job not long ago, but I am currently looking for a better one. I feel independent and capable of managing myself and my anxiety. I am going to the gym and grocery stores all by myself without any worry.

IMMEDIATE SUGGESTIONS FOR PEOPLE WHO IDENTIFY WITH SOME PARTS OF OFELIA'S STORY

Disclaimer: Mental health and addiction issues should not be addressed alone. Please seek professional help to reach the highest level of emotional well-being possible. These suggestions can be used as support for professional help or for people who are not suffering as seriously as XXX.

1. **Self-soothing Technique – Distraction.** Distraction is a very effective technique for changing your mood. Distraction interrupts your negative mood by engaging in something that distracts you from what has upset you. It is that simple. The way it works is that when you realized you have become upset and are unable to process it quickly and return to peace of mind you should enact this technique. Everyone is different and the following activities will not apply to everyone but hopefully you will either see one you enjoy or you may have already thought of one for yourself. Here are some examples:
    a. Watching a movie or streaming a show,
    b. Reading a book
    c. Dancing
    d. Listening to music
    e. Exercising
    f. Cleaning your house
    g. Organizing a room in your house
    h. Surfing the net
    i. Write or journal
    j. Sing
    k. (Insert your own here)
    Whichever activity you choose, it must be one you like and that you can do for about 30 minutes.

2. **Positive Affirmations** – Affirmations are positive messages we give ourselves to change the way we think or feel about ourselves or our behavior. Once you recognize an area of your life you would like to change an affirmation can help you change that. It is very simple. For example, if I want to

increase my self-esteem I can say "I am a smart, caring, giving person'. By repeating this phrase I am building the confidence I need to behave the way I feel I should behave, in this example, **confident.**

When practicing affirmations, choose one or two to focus on for several weeks. Say the affirmation out loud in a confident voice several times a day and before you go to bed. (Bonus hint: Say your affirmation out loud while standing in front of a mirror)

3. **Exercise** – Many studies confirm what we have heard for many years. Exercise is essential, it benefits our physical and emotional needs to have a healthy, active life. But for so many of us, especially if we are suffering from depression, getting started is very difficult. These five steps on how to get started are from Live Science.
    a. **Be Safe** – Safety first. You should never begin an exercise program before checking with your doctor. If you have a health condition, speak with your doctor about whether you'll need to take any precautions when you exercise.
    b. **Enjoy yourself** – Pick an exercise that you enjoy doing. This could be a more traditional form of exercise, like jogging or going to the gym; sports like tennis or soccer; or even a dance class.
    c. **Start Gradually** – Start out with a fairly light activity, and gradually increase the duration and intensity of exercise. The goal is to complete 30 minutes of exercise a day, five days a week. These 30 minutes can be done all at once, or broken up into 10-minute increments.
    d. **Don't Overdo it** – Avoid high-impact exercises, which involve lots of jumping or ballistic movements, because these can lead to injury when you are first starting out.
    e. **Set goals** – Set goals to keep yourself motivated in your exercise, like running a 5K or improving your time. You might also consider getting a friend to exercise with you to hold you accountable.

Chapter 7

Johnny's solution to Substance Use Disorder and Oppositional Defiant Disorder

Our son had a 3-year history of daily use of marijuana and alcohol. Johnny has been suspended from school, lies, and has been involved with gangs and in firearm possession. He was once shot in the leg, he said it was an accident but he had left very little room for us to believe him. Our son was oppositional and defiant with authority figures at home and at school.

Prior to using alcohol and drugs, our son was active and loved to play soccer, but soon after his drug abuse started he left these behind, he does not play soccer anymore.

Johnny, our son, is 15-years-old and we brought him to counseling due to his drinking and marijuana use. He is also showing some signs of depression. Johnny was born in the United States, in Atlanta, Georgia, but we, his parents, are from Mexico and feel very strong about our roots and our heritage. Johnny was hospitalized last week because of a suicide attempt while he was drinking and using drugs. At first, he told us that he had cut himself on a window but we know better. When he drinks, Johnny becomes aggressive toward us, his brother, and himself. Our son had been arrested for smoking marijuana and skipping school in the past. He has also been suspended for skipping school and for fighting, despite all of this his grades usually average around a 'C'.

There has been no history of any kind of mental illness in our family but there is a strong history of substance abuse.

Our son doesn't open his heart to us very much anymore, but occasionally, he does share some things when he is troubled a lot. He once told us that he felt sad and depressed in the past and had previously thought about suicide. He told us that he doesn't have any suicidal or homicidal ideation at this time, after the hospital. When we came in seeking help, the counselors asked Johnny signed a safety plan they had developed, and he did.

Johnny seemed to be willing to cooperate with the counselors and would very likely go along with the treatment. This made us very happy. Johnny was guarded but cooperative but we were told that was expected. Johnny showed symptoms that meet the diagnosis for Alcohol abuse, Cannabis abuse and Oppositional Defiant Disorder.

Johnny was assigned a counselor who specialized in adolescents, he was assigned to attend a substance abuse group and to participate in social and support activities at the clinic with other young people with similar problems. We were invited to participate in the family program.

The plan was for Johnny to learn new skills and new things to do so he would not want to drink alcohol and use marijuana, to learn how to process the things he liked to do against the use of drugs and the consequences of using drugs.

We were given a list of places to connect Johnny with neighborhood activities and organizations; tutoring was also provided to Johnny. A setting was created to facilitate discussions and activities around living a drug-free life. We began to attend family counseling to process with the family the events in Johnny's life in order to help us be supportive and provide him with the opportunity to regain trust.

Small but important and achievable goals were set out for our son, he was to decrease or stop using alcohol and marijuana at whatever pace was easy for him, improve grades to a B average, identify three ways in which drinking and smoking marijuana has negatively affected him and his school work, learn three coping strategies (playing sports, calling a friend for support, listening to music) to prevent him from smoking marijuana or using alcohol and attempt to make at least two supportive friends who do not influence him to use substances.

Part of how the family played a role was by having dinner together nightly instead of isolating. To increase his ability to communicate his feelings, Johnny was asked to express at least one his emotions to his mother three times a week.

Johnny worked on identifying two to four thoughts that trigger his sadness that leads to suicidal thoughts and write them down to discuss with the therapists and to begin to practice the coping skills and the refusal skills he was learning so it becomes easier to avoid situations with alcohol or drugs.

After treatment, Johnny is still struggling with school but has made moderate improvement and had begun to use some new studying skills. He plans to continue with the tutoring services. He no longer feels suicidal. Our son has not had any incidents with drinking or using drugs and he has not made any suicidal statements. He is still having problems managing his emotions but we understand that this is a process and we all must continue to be patient.

IMMEDIATE SUGGESTIONS FOR PEOPLE WHO IDENTIFY WITH SOME PARTS OF JOHNNY'S STORY

Disclaimer: Mental health and addiction issues should not be addressed alone. Please seek professional help to reach the highest level of emotional well-being possible. These suggestions can be used as support for professional help or for people who are not suffering as seriously as Johnny.

1. **Parents - Seek Professional Help:** Helping an adolescent who is struggling with substance abuse and/or a mental health issue is not easy. The mental health of the entire family is affected when one member is having difficulties, especially if that member is a child. Mental health is very valuable and we should not deny ourselves and our families the gift of being happy and being able to function fully in our lives with everything we want to do. To find help, you can go to https://findtreatment.samhsa.gov/
2. **Tutoring** – This service is one of the most beneficial services to help youth who are experimenting with alcohol, drugs and other risky behaviors and who are having academic difficulty. Often young people will use alcohol and drugs because they are bored. But many times that translates to "I don't know how to study and am doing poorly I school, therefore I will use alcohol and drugs." But, in my experience, once we empower them academically, they soar and the risky behaviors tend to rapidly decrease and even stop. There are many types of tutoring, peer tutors (by other students), professional tutors, in-home tutors, on-line tutors, and others. Tutoring is helping students improve their learning strategies in order to promote independence and empowerment. The purpose of tutoring is to help students help themselves, assisting them to become independent learners and thus no longer needing a tutor.
3. **Visualization** – This is one of the Cognitive Behavioral Therapy Techniques often used by clinicians. Visualization is simply rehearsing in your mind where you want to see yourself, typically for about five minutes each day. Then you just repeat the images over and over again. With visualization you use your mind and your imagination to create images of having achieved

your goal. For example, Johnny would visualize getting a B on his test; playing soccer again; not using alcohol and drugs; and others. When visualizing you always want to visualize that you already have the thing you want.

Chapter 8

Alana's solution to Depression and Post Traumatic Stress Disorder

I was feeling depressed since the beginning of this year. I had a history of depression beginning eight years ago, when it got so bad that I even thought about suicide. Back then, I was diagnosed with postpartum depression when I gave birth to my daughter.

I am a 44-year-old woman originally from Acapulco, Mexico. I first decided to seek help in part due to feeling very guilty about having stayed in a domestic violent relationship with my husband. For a while I was a victim of domestic violence, including physical abuse once, and repeated verbal and emotional abuse from my husband. We have been together for the last 19 years and married for 16 years. The abuse started 16 years ago, just after our marriage, when I told him that I was pregnant with his child he asked me to have an abortion but I had no plan of doing such a thing. I decided to leave him a few years ago but he developed a heart condition and thus I decided to stay with him, it is not easy to break bonds developed in 16 years. I thought he would change, but he didn't, I was wrong. I have decided, it is the time to get divorced, but I don't know how to do it. I rarely have any contact with my husband even though we are living in the same house, we stay in separate rooms.

When I announced my decision to leave him, he decided to strike back by telling our kids that I wanted to abandon him, and that I have

Alana's solution to Depression and Post Traumatic Stress Disorder

been unfaithful which is a total lie, how can someone lie like that? Or make such accusations without any proof? I was sad about the situation and the way he was talking about me to our kids. It's not just me he has also been emotionally abusive to our kids too.

Most of the time my sleep is normal. The sense of guilt for not leaving my husband when my kids were little and is worse than anyone can ever imagine. Feelings of hopelessness and worthlessness were part of my routine.

Over the course of time my appetite has decreased which I believe also caused lack of motivation, energy and concentration. Soon after that I started losing interest in doing things that usually brought me pleasure. Our children know better and they are supportive of the divorce, they tell me that one of them can stay to help their dad with his medical issues if I decided to leave him.

Getting anxious and worried about your children is a part of a mother's job, and I am no different, I have been excessively worried about my son getting in trouble, I suspect he is probably smoking marijuana and drinking. I get so worried and anxious that I fear I will have a panic attack, that is something that has never happened and I hope it never happens in the future. I was afraid that my husband would do something to me although he never made any threats. There was a state of fear and anxiety in the house.

I am a pretty healthy person, and I have not had any medical problems, never have I done anything to end up in a hospital, I'm not on any medications, I don't not drink, use drugs or smoke. There have been cases of substance abuse in my family.

In the past, I was able to work menial jobs but nothing steady. I'm currently studying to complete my requirements to obtain a high school equivalency diploma or GED (General Educational Development).

When I was admitted for counseling, I was open and honest with the staff and was somewhat excited but also fearful about what would come next.

I was told I had post-traumatic stress disorder (PTSD) and depression. I was assigned a counselor for individual therapy and began to see a psychiatrist for medication to help me get better.

I feel lucky that I was helped by such great people, they provided me with a lot of information about domestic violence, how to improve my self-esteem, assertiveness, and co-dependency in a group setting.

They educated me about the cycle of domestic violence and how to break that cycle. I was given training and was helped in developing a domestic violence safety plan.

My interpersonal skills got better, even more than I could ever have done it on my own. During the time I was in counseling they helped me identify feelings, thoughts and events that may be contributing to unhealthy communication with my children. But they also showed me what to do to improve communication with my children. I also improved quality interactions with my children.

I could identify behaviors in my family that were harmful and how to correct them. They also helped me prepare physically, financially and emotionally to file for divorce.

I was discharged with the confidence that I have learned a lot about domestic violence and about the safety strategies that I need. I now feel strong enough mentally, physically and spiritually and I have also filed divorce. I learned new interpersonal skills to take care of my emotions and I learned new strategies and the quality of my interactions with my children have improved dramatically. I have almost completed my GED preparation, and I will be taking the exam soon.

IMMEDIATE SUGGESTIONS FOR PEOPLE WHO IDENTIFY WITH SOME PARTS OF ALANA'S STORY

Disclaimer: Mental health and addiction issues should not be addressed alone. Please seek professional help to reach the highest level of emotional well-being possible. These suggestions can be used as support for professional help or for people who are not suffering as seriously as Alana.
<u>Domestic violence, or intimate partner violence</u>, *is a willful single occurrence or a pattern of abusive behavior employing coercion, threat, intimidation, isolation, power or fear that results in physical, psychological or emotional trauma. Family violence is never acceptable.*

1. **EMPOWERMENT APPROACH**- Empowerment theory underpins services provided by many clinics, shelters, and nonprofit organizations. This approach is grounded in the belief that victims of domestic violence should have access to information, education, and other necessary social and economic support to make informed decisions that best reflect their interests and needs. Rather than attempting to eliminate the violence, which is not controlled by victims, the empowerment approach uses knowledge dissemination, training, and counseling to create a set of services that victims control, such as post-victimization assistance and risk minimization. In Alana's case, Alana was receiving tools to empower her in how she communicates, how she acts and how she functions. By completing her GED she was being empowered to be able to apply for and acquire better job opportunities. Family violence Hotline 1-800-799-7233 ; http://www.thehotline.org
2. Use of 'I' Statements – In order to minimize blame and to improve how we can communicate our feelings clearly, therapists often recommend the use of 'I' statements. Usually an 'I' statement is followed by 'when you'. This way we can ensure that we are focusing on the issue, the behavior, and not the person. For example, "**I feel** hurt **when you** forgot out date because it makes it look like you don't care about our relationship". 'I' statements are <u>assertive</u> and not <u>aggressive.</u> You can create your own 'I' statements by first writing down

how you would have said something and then changing it into an 'I..when you..' statement. In our example above, the initial statement could have been "You made me so angry because you forgot our date." Here the focus is on the person, "**You** made me ..." Whereas when you say "**I feel** hurt **when you** forgot out date because it makes it look like you don't care about our relationship", you are focusing on the feeling (hurt) and the action (forgot our date) and not the person.

Chapter 9

Laura's solution to Depression and Anxiety

I have had a history of trauma. I was raped by my uncle when I was seven years old and repeatedly raped by my cousin from the ages of 8-14. I was involved in a physically, emotionally, and verbally abusive marriage for nine years until it ended. My current husband is no prince charming. He is jealous and controlling. He lied when we were dating. I later found out that he was married and had kids in his country, but even after I found that out, I decided to stay with him.

I am Laura, a 35-year-old woman from Mexico City, Mexico. My story is about overcoming depression. I would often get depressed, and I didn't know what to do. I was having trouble sleeping and was not eating very much, I just was not hungry. Maybe all of this was happening because I was going through a separation with my husband and it had been very stressful for me. During this time I started having very little energy and started missing days of work. I was easily irritated, and I felt anxious about everything almost every day. I experienced panic attacks in the past. Once, I got aggressive with my husband and threw a chair at him but that was the only time I became aggressive.

I was traumatized when I found out that my daughter was molested by my nephew for several years. How could I have been so blind? I felt a lot of guilt about my daughter being molested. I wish I was able to protect her. I wish I was able to save my daughter and shield her from what I have been through.

I admit that I have had thoughts of suicide and of wanting to die in the past. I sometimes drive carelessly when I am by myself. But no matter how bad my life got, I never planned or intended to harm myself or any others.

I live with my three children, a 17-year-old daughter, an 11-year-old daughter, and a one-year-old son. My relationship with my oldest daughter is not very good. My oldest daughter is rebellious, more than you can imagine, and we fight all the time. Other than that I have a good relationship with my other children.

I was born in a large family; I am the fifth child out of eight siblings. I had a very close relationship with my father who was overprotective and very affectionate, but I was never able to have a close relationship with mother. My mother was very strict and would often beat me.

I first got married at the age of 17 to a man who was physically, verbally, and sexually abusive. I immigrated to the U.S. at the age of 25, saved money for two years and was able to bring my children to join me. I divorced my first husband at the age of 28, and 3 months later, I became involved in my second relationship. I married my second husband 8 months ago.

I enjoy a good social life with three close friends who are very supportive. I enjoy reading, going out with my children, and shopping. I finished the 6th grade of school but did not go any further. I work as a babysitter, a waitress at a night club, and currently, I cleans houses.

I have always been a law-abiding person and the only medical problem that I had, if I remember correctly, was a concussion when my first husband hit me. Recently, I was told that I have some problem with my kidneys.

I've had a history of depression and sadness, of being unhappy. And finally I am seeking help. In Mexico the only places I ever heard of for mental health help were big psychiatric hospitals, but that used to scare me so I never went there.

I was glad to be getting help. I usually don't want to admit I have problems and either ignore them or make them look like they are not serious or important. This led to my delay in getting help for many years. I am always saying 'it's not that bad' or 'it will be better tomorrow.' But then I was here, telling my story to professionals in hopes that they could help me live a better life, improve my relationship with my children and feel better about myself.

I was told that I was suffering from depression and anxiety and that I was not alone. That made me feel better. I started seeing a wonderful counselor for individual sessions, another counselor for a group with other women with similar problems and the doctor who gave me medication for depression and anxiety.

My counseling also included new tools to help me be a better parent. I needed to identify between two and three strategies I used to parent my children so we could work on those to make them better or improve their behavior. I was taught skills to be a better mother, like encouraging my children, setting boundaries, install logical consequences and understanding my children's needs.

I also identified triggers for my anger and I explored new ways of reacting to anger differently than in the past. I learned many new skills like tolerance and how to communicate better. I learned relaxation exercises like deep breathing and muscle relaxation. Against all the odds, the results were more effective than I had ever imagined.

I started talking to my children calmly within six months. I started using strategies that I learned to parent my children. I wasn't afraid of being alone, I reduced my fears and increased social interactions with family and friends, but working thing things out with my husband will take a little more time. I also started to control my impulsivity.

Just like I mentioned before, after six months, I began to communicate better as I worked to become more independent. I was able to use the skills I learned to calm myself, to think through my thoughts before I give an answer, and to speak confidently. I was able to follow through on my decisions.

I also found myself being more focused during my English classes.

Now, I am hopeful that with new skills I will be able to be more independent and have more options to manage my feelings when upset or fearful. I feel less dependent on others and that I consider a personal achievement. I don't fight with my husband as much as I used to, but I know that I still need to improve my communication skills. I have begun to talk more with my older daughter and to express love as I should. This is how it is all supposed to be. Things will get even better with time; I know they will.

IMMIDIATE SUGGESTIONS FOR PEOPLE WHO IDENTIFY WITH SOME PARTS OF LAURA'S STORY

Disclaimer: Mental health and addiction issues should not be addressed alone. Please seek professional help to reach the highest level of emotional well-being possible. These suggestions can be used as support for professional help or for people who are not suffering as seriously as Laura's.

1. **Practice Anger Management Skills** – I recommend these tips published by the Mayo Clinic staff https://www.mayoclinic.org/healthy-lifestyle/adult-health/in-depth/anger-management/art-20045434?pg=1

   i. **Think before you speak**
   In the heat of the moment, it's easy to say something you'll later regret. Take a few moments to collect your thoughts before saying anything — and allow others involved in the situation to do the same.

   ii. **Once you're calm, express your anger**
   As soon as you're thinking clearly, express your frustration in an assertive but non-confrontational way. State your concerns and needs clearly and directly, without hurting others or trying to control them.

   iii. **Get some exercise**
   Physical activity can help reduce stress that can cause you to become angry. If you feel your anger escalating, go for a brisk walk or run, or spend some time doing other enjoyable physical activities.

   iv. **Take a timeout**
   Timeouts aren't just for kids. Give yourself short breaks during times of the day that tend to be stressful. A few moments of quiet time might help you feel better prepared to handle what's ahead without getting irritated or angry.

   v. **Identify possible solutions**
   Instead of focusing on what made you mad, work on resolving the issue at hand. Does your child's messy room drive you crazy? Close the door. Is your partner late for

dinner every night? Schedule meals later in the evening — or agree to eat on your own a few times a week. Remind yourself that anger won't fix anything and might only make it worse.

vi. **Stick with 'I' statements**
To avoid criticizing or placing blame — which might only increase tension — use "I" statements to describe the problem. Be respectful and specific. For example, say, "I'm upset that you left the table without offering to help with the dishes" instead of "You never do any housework."

vii. **Don't hold a grudge**
Forgiveness is a powerful tool. If you allow anger and other negative feelings to crowd out positive feelings, you might find yourself swallowed up by your own bitterness or sense of injustice. But if you can forgive someone who angered you, you might both learn from the situation and strengthen your relationship.

viii. **Use humor to release tension**
Lightening up can help diffuse tension. Use humor to help you face what's making you angry and, possibly, any unrealistic expectations you have for how things should go. Avoid sarcasm, though — it can hurt feelings and make things worse.

ix. **Practice relaxation skills**
When your temper flares, put relaxation skills to work. Practice deep-breathing exercises, imagine a relaxing scene, or repeat a calming word or phrase, such as "Take it easy." You might also listen to music, write in a journal or do a few yoga poses — whatever it takes to encourage relaxation.

x. **Know when to seek help**
Learning to control anger is a challenge for everyone at times. Seek help for anger issues if your anger seems out of control, causes you to do things you regret or hurts those around you.

2. **Setting boundaries** – A boundary is a rule, a guide that you can create to let other people know what behavior is acceptable to you so they know how you would expect them to behave.

For example, for Laura, a boundary may be to let her romantic partners that she will not tolerate any type of physical or emotional violence. To set your own boundaries you must look within yourself and find out what is important to you, why you would set that boundary and what you are willing to do if someone chooses to violate the boundary you have set.

3. **Deep Breathing Technique** - The 4-7-8 Exercise

    The 4-7-8 breathing exercise is very simple, it can be done anywhere, and you can do it at any time. The 4-7-8 breathing technique, championed by practitioner and teacher of integrative medicine Andrew Weill, is simple and worth trying. It's free, quick and doesn't require equipment.

    Before you begin, sit with your back straight and place the tip of your tongue on the roof of your mouth just above your teeth and keep it there throughout the exercise.

    - Exhale completely through your mouth - quite forcefully so you make a "whoosh" sound.
    - Close your mouth and inhale quietly and softly through your nose for a mental count of **four.**
    - Hold your breath and count to **seven.**
    - Exhale completely through your mouth, making another whoosh sound for **eight** seconds in one large breath.
    - Inhale again and repeat the cycle three times for a total of four breaths.

Remember: All inhaling breaths must be quiet and through your nose and all exhaling breaths must be loud and through your mouth.

Chapter 10

Roberto's solution for Schizophrenia

I am Roberto, and I am 24 years old. I voluntarily sought mental health treatment. I came to the clinic with my brother Gonzalo; I wasn't able to communicate very well at that time, more like I didn't want to, my brother did all the talking for me. I had been previously diagnosed with schizophrenia, psychosis and mild intellectual disability, after that I went to live in Perú for a few years.

I was born and raised in Perú by my parents and I moved to the United States in order to live with my older brother when I was 13 years old. I was bullied a lot in school when I was 14 years old while living in California. I first realized that I speak to myself during that time and for that, I was hospitalized for one month. After that, I went back to Perú to live with my mother, and I never went back to school again. I was seeing a psychiatrist every three months and have been taking medication regularly. I always felt lucky that I was able to find a psychiatrist and other professionals in Perú; depending on where you live some mental health services are available.

There has been no history of alcohol, illicit drug use in my family, but mental health problems are another story. I have two cousins who suffer from trichinosis, a parasitic disease, and then they were diagnosed with schizophrenia. Another cousin from mother's side has been diagnosed with autism, and my sister's nephew also suffers from autism.

My father was never home and had other relationships. I am the youngest, and my mother had me when she was 45 years old, she passed away when I was 23 and that was when I moved back to the United States once again.

Now I am back in the United States and I wanted to continue to receive medication and treatment because I was hearing voices in my head every day. I live with my older brother and his family. I asked him to make an appointment for me and he took me for an evaluation.

I was withdrawn during the interview as it was very difficult for me to process anything that they asked me at that time.

The only talking I did while I was in the counselor's office the first time, was with my brother and it was more like whispering than talking. I was having trouble concentrating during the whole session. I wasn't able to recall information to answer questions, but, I was able to recall some stuff with the help of my brother. It was difficult for me to answer any of the questions that were asked, it was taking a lot of time for me to process what they were asking. I realized that I was looking down a lot while trying to make sense of the situation. I would sometimes talk to myself and since, at times, I am distrustful of others, I didn't speak too much in the session. I also wasn't able to complete my evaluation without my brother's assistance.

My brother told me that the counselor who was evaluating me shared how he saw me during the evaluation, it sounded something like this: *"During the evaluation, when asked where he was, Roberto reported that he was at doctor's office. Roberto couldn't report the time or situation; his mood was blunted, dull and bland. He had a flat affect. His attitude towards interviewer was suspicious, guarded and evasive. He denies the presence of problems in his life. Roberto has an impaired ability to make routine decisions; his memory is remote and he has difficulty processing information. Roberto is well groomed and clean, his manner of dress is age appropriate, his posture was slumped; his speech slow and his content was appropriate."* It sounded so weird to hear that but when they explained it to me it made sense, I usually slump, don't like to answer questions and stay quiet.

I suffered from paranoia and heard voices during the interview that told me "someday I will die." I also sometimes feel that bugs are crawling all over, something called tactile hallucinations. There were also times when I would scratch my skin at night so much that I would get scabs from it. I used to think to myself that I want to have a better life. I was also a much-reserved person I did not communicate anything not even when was sick.

I used to talk to myself as if I was talking to someone else on a daily basis. I also had the fear I was always being chased. I was very forgetful and forget to do things unless reminded.

I do realize that sometimes I get irritable and yell at my niece and nephew, but I have never gotten aggressive. I don't have any friends. I spend my time with my brother Gonzalo and his family but I don't talk to them much.

I have a daily routine and am usually good at following directions. Even though I hurt myself at times with the scratching I never had any ideations or intentions of suicide. It is a dream of mine to find a job and have a normal routine. I would love to be able to be more active and be part of my family's life, and for that, I continue taking medication and continue to work on improving my communication skills.

Things are a little better now. I need to remember that the counselors told me that recovery is a journey and I may have good days and bad days. I have to remember that I need to find the things that help me feel better and help me maintain wellness.

I was supposed to see my counselor two to three times a week to start, but sometimes I did not feel up to going. When I did go I liked it. She helped me understand the illness I had and reminded me that I have had good periods of health and wellness before. And that I can get there again. I went to counseling on and off for about one year and it did help me.

When I finished my sessions my family members told the counselors that I was calmer and that I reported fewer hallucinations and was more stable. They told them that I was also now able to take my medication on my own and was also helping out with some chores at home and was better at doing things for myself.

I may go back to Perú.

IMMEDIATE SUGGESTIONS FOR PEOPLE WHO IDENTIFY WITH SOME PARTS OF ROBERTO's STORY

Disclaimer: Mental health and addiction issues should not be addressed alone. Please seek professional help to reach the highest level of emotional well-being possible. These suggestions can be used as support for professional help or for people who are not suffering as seriously as Roberto.

There are several places to go to find methods to support your own recovery and for the family and friends to help support you in your recovery. One place is https://www.mentalhealth.gov/basics/recovery/index.html.

I want to offer two sets of suggestions, one set for the individual and one set for their friends and families.

FOR THE INDIVIDUAL:

1. **Take the lead role of managing your own recovery** – Today there is a very strong consumer movement that has made a tremendous amount of progress in helping individuals with a mental illness take charge and make decisions about their recovery. There are several certification programs that will help the individual and some programs that will allow that individual to help others.
2. **Set attainable goals** – For individuals seeking recovery and wellness, it is important to set goals that will guarantee positive results. These can include things like engaging in meaningful daily activities, such as a job or school, volunteering, caring for your family, or being creative. Work for independence, income, and resources to participate in society.

FOR FRIENDS AND FAMILY:

1. **Be an Advocate:** To help someone have a successful recovery experience we must become advocates and help them speak up when they can't. In this story, I mentioned that Roberto's brother, Gonzalo, had to speak for Roberto during interviews and sessions in order for the team of professionals could understand Roberto's struggles and

successes and provide the help he needed. Once Roberto could speak for himself, his brother stepped back.
2. **Help them comply with their treatment** – This can be as simple as helping them check their daily list; be there to listen; providing rides to the doctor or pharmacy; in short being there for when the person needs support.
3. **Offer emotional support and encouragement** – A person can sometimes feel disorganized and hearing the encouragement of family and friends can be very beneficial.

Appendix

Definition of Counseling Services Mentioned in this Book

Individual Counseling: Individual counseling or therapy is a process through which clients work one-on-one with a trained therapist to address their mental health or substance use disorder problems. Sessions are structured and time limited to 60 or sometimes 90 minutes. Clients are guided through clinical techniques to explore their behaviors, beliefs and feelings and create a plan to change those areas of their lives that are creating conflict. The length of time someone receives individual counseling depends on several factors including the presenting problems, supports available to achieve goals and the client's ability to change.

Group Counseling: Group counseling involves a small group, usually no more than 12 individuals, who frequently meet with a trained therapist to work on interpersonal relationships and address common issues shared by the members. Some groups are open ended which means there is no beginning or end and clients come in and out of the group as they achieve their goals. Other groups are very specific and address an issue for a fixed period; these may include trauma groups, Attention Deficit Disorder Group and others.

Nursing Services: The nursing services include laboratory analysis, tuberculosis (TB) testing, drug testing and voluntary HIV/AIDS testing. Nursing services also include educating clients on psychotropic and other medications and lifestyle and nutritional issues that may be affecting their well-being. The nurse also provides the testing necessary before a client is placed on psychotropic medications.

Psychiatric Services: A staff psychiatrist provides a Diagnostic Assessment, Medication Management and Medication follow up services.

Recovery Support Services: These services are out-of-office services that provide support to the individual between counseling sessions. They include home or school visits to see how the client is functioning and to help clients who may be struggling in achieving their treatment goals.

Dr. Mancini's recommended assessment tools

Screening tools for depression, anxiety and posttraumatic stress disorder (PTSD) for ADULTS:

- Patient Health Questionnaire-9 (PHQ-9) - The PHQ-9 is a concise, self-administered tool for assessing depression. It is a free and publically available tool that can be downloaded in 30 different languages at http://www.phqscreeners.com/. The manual and scoring guide are available at: https://phqscreeners.pfizer.edrupalgardens.com/sites/g/files/g10016261/f/201412/instructions.pdf.
  Reference information for the utility of the PHQ-9 for the assessment of depression can be found at http://www.apa.org/pi/about/publications/caregivers/practice-settings/assessment/tools/patient-health.aspx.
- Generalized Anxiety Disorder-7 item scale (GAD-7) is a screening tool for generalized anxiety disorder which identifies whether a complete assessment for anxiety is indicated.[1] It is a free and publically available tool that can be downloaded in 30 different languages at http://www.phqscreeners.com/.
- The Primary Care PTSD Screen (PC-PTSD) is a 4-item screen that was designed for use in primary care and other medical settings for the identification of posttraumatic stress disorder. This tool and its instructions are available at http://www.ptsd.va.gov/professional/assessment/screens/pc-ptsd.asp.

Screening tools for depression and psychosocial problems in CHILDREN/ADOLESCENTS:

- The Pediatric Symptom Checklist-17 (PSC-17) (parent/caretaker version) is a brief screening questionnaire that is used by pediatricians and other health professionals to improve the recognition and treatment of psychosocial problems in children ages 4 to 18 years old. This tool is available over 12 languages and is publically available at http://www.massgeneral.org/psychiatry/services/psc_home.aspx.

---

[1] Source: Spitzer RL, Kroenke K, Williams JBW, Lowe B. A brief measure for assessing generalized anxiety disorder. Arch Inern Med. 2006;166:1092-1097.

Patient Health Questionnaire-Adolescent (PHQ-A) - The PHQ-A was adapted from the PHQ-9 modified for Adolescents (PHQ-A)[2], which is in the public domain (http://www.phqscreeners.com/instructions/instructions.pdf). The PHQ-A is a concise, self-administered tool for assessing depression in children ages 12-18 years old. It is a free and publically available at http://www.ohsu.edu/xd/education/schools/school-of-medicine/departments/clinical-departments/psychiatry/divisions-and-clinics/child-and-adolescent-psychiatry/opal-k/upload/PHQ-A-Severity-Measure-for-Depression.pdf

---

[2] The reference for the original measure is: Johnson JG, Harris ES, Spitzer RL, Williams JBW: The Patient Health Questionnaire for Adolescents: Validation of an instrument for the assessment of mental disorders among adolescent primary care patients. J Adolescent Health 30:196–204, 2002.

www.ingramcontent.com/pod-product-compliance
Lightning Source LLC
Chambersburg PA
CBHW070212230526

45471CB00002B/933